Angel in Blue
The Story of Ashley Martin

Angel in Blue

The Story of Ashley Martin

Written and illustrated by fifth-grade students of
Smith Road Elementary School in Temperance, Michigan

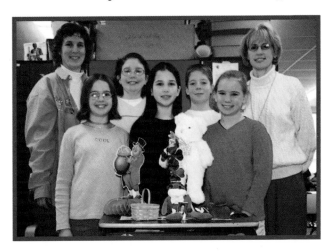

Meet the Authors, Friends of Ashley:
L-R: Jenny Haley, Katie Oldaker, Nicole Gin, T.J. Ward (illustrator), and Alaina Kirk
Advisors: Margaret Spoelman and Thea Kirkwood

SCHOLASTIC INC.
New York   Toronto   London   Auckland   Sydney
Mexico City   New Delhi   Hong Kong

Copyright © 2000 by Scholastic Inc.
All rights reserved. Published by Scholastic Inc.
SCHOLASTIC and associated logos are trademarks and/or registered trademarks of Scholastic Inc.

ISBN 0-439-26065-5

12 11 10 9 8 7 6 5 4 3   00 01 02 03 04

Printed in the U.S.A.   08
First printing, October 2000

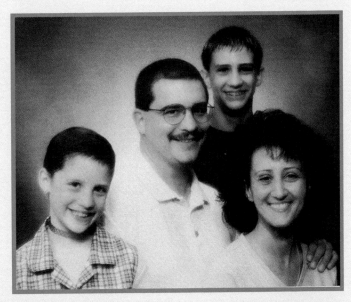

L-R: Ashley, Keith, Kris, and Carolyn Martin

This book is dedicated to the Martin family, especially to Ashley's dad who said, "If you are going to write a book about Ashley, be sure to make it BLUE!"

We are writing this book because we miss Ashley and we want you to try to live your life as Ashley did.

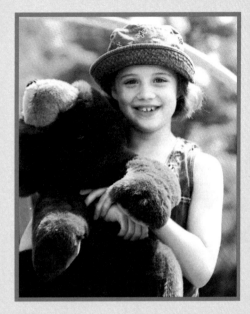

ABOUT ASHLEY…

This is a book. Well, of course it's a book, but this is a *special* book about a *special* girl named Ashley. She had a type of cancer called rhabdomyosarcoma. It is a rare cancer that most often affects children between the ages of six and ten.

You will see the words "Ashley says…" at the bottom of each spread. When you turn the page you will see a message from Ashley.

We chose the BLUE theme because BLUE was Ashley's favorite color…. We don't want to give too much away, so read on to hear Ashley's story.

How do you pronounce rhabdomyosarcoma?
Ashley Martin didn't know the answer either until
she was diagnosed with this rare form of cancer.
Ashley's mom and dad took her to the doctor after
finding a big bump above her ankle. She was
only eight.

How would you feel if you were diagnosed with cancer?

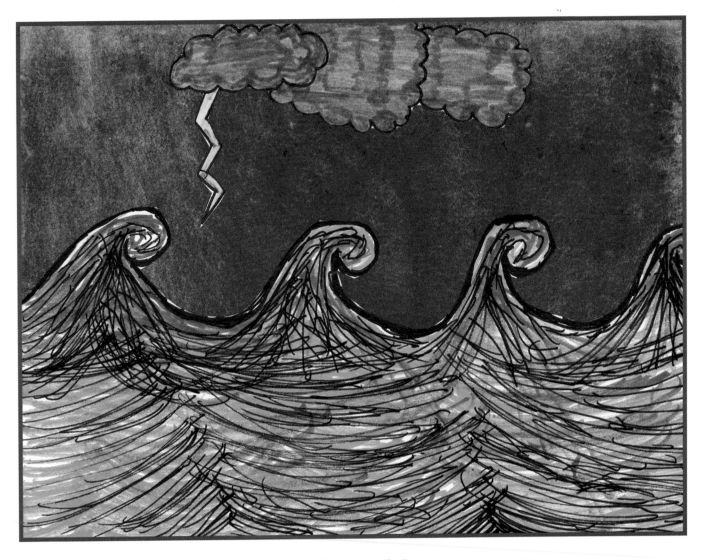

Sometimes Ashley felt as blue as a stormy sea.

Ashley says . . .

" . . . Laugh a little, Giggle a lot! "

When Ashley laughed it was pretty funny. Her friends couldn't help laughing along with her, even if they didn't get the joke.

How would it feel to laugh when you're sick?

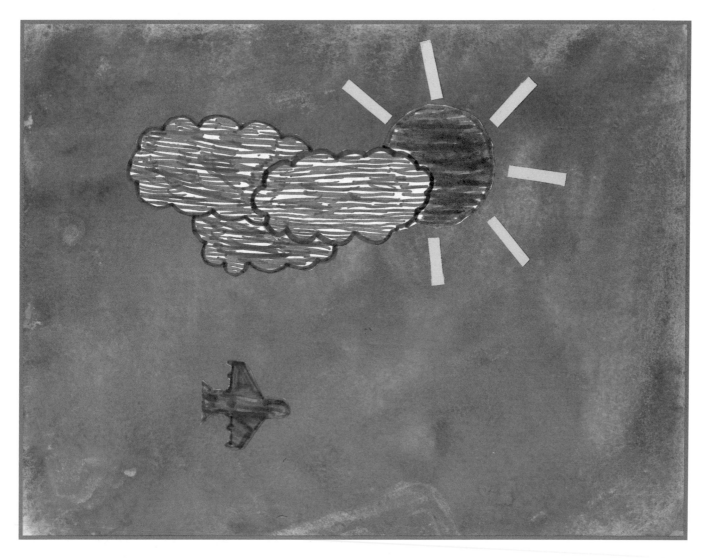

Sometimes Ashley felt as blue as a sunny sky.

Ashley says . . .

" . . . Don't take your health for granted! "

Having cancer meant Ashley had to visit the doctor and the hospital a lot. One time she was in the hospital for a bone marrow transplant operation. Her teacher, Mrs. Tompkins, helped her to plan a birthday party for her dad. It was a surprise party. The doctors and nurses all helped them celebrate his birthday in her hospital room. They called it "a birthday in a box."

How would you feel if you were in the hospital on your dad's birthday?

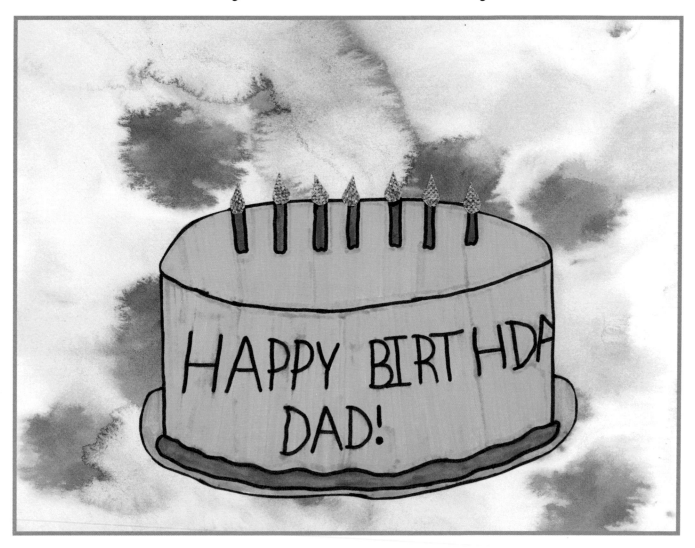

Sometimes Ashley felt as blue as frosting on a birthday cake.

Ashley says . . .

" ... Having cancer stinks! "

Ashley loved school, but she had to miss more class-
es than she wanted. Most days she had to leave
before lunch to go have chemotherapy. If she couldn't
make up her work, she didn't have to! Ashley was
lucky because her teachers were her tutors.

How would you feel if you HAD to stay home?

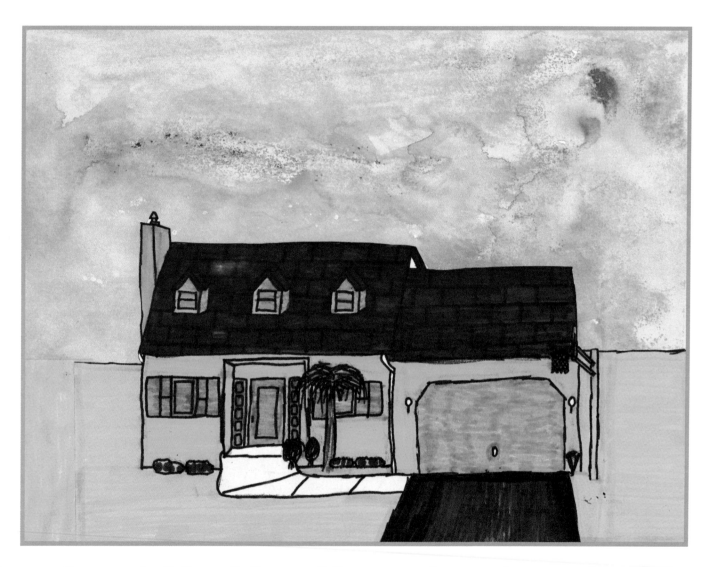

Sometimes Ashley felt as blue as the paint on her house.

Ashley says . . .

" . . . Spend as much time as you can with your friends! "

Nobody was a better friend to anyone than Ashley. She had a ton of friends. Her friends cared about her and she cared about them. People were always trying to find ways to help her.

How would you feel if you didn't get to see your friends as much as you wanted?

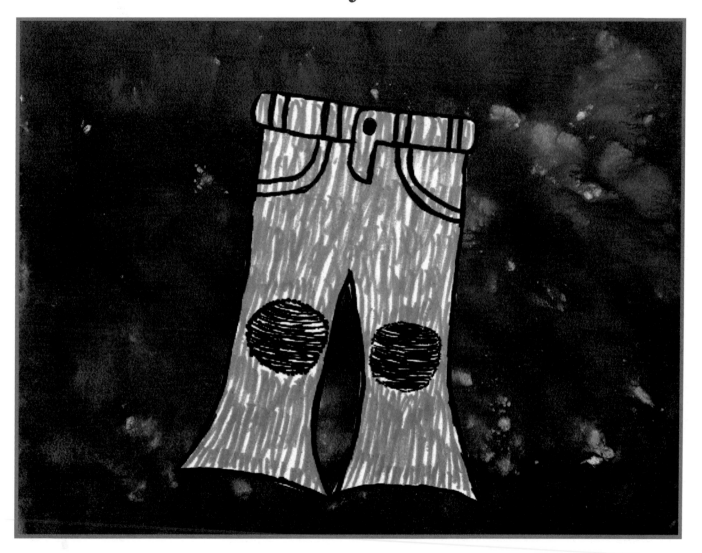

Sometimes Ashley felt as blue as faded jeans.

Ashley says . . .

" . . . Remember to tell your friends thank you! "

One of the ways people in the community helped Ashley was to participate in a benefit sponsored by the school. It was called the "Beanie Baby Benefit." The goal was to collect one thousand Beanie Babies and sell them at a silent auction to raise "Martin Money" for Ashley. If the school collected one thousand Beanie Babies, the gym teacher would shave his head!

They more than met this goal, and the school raised over $26,000!! So, Ashley got to shave the gym teacher's head! It was very cool.

How would you feel if your school pulled together a benefit just for you?

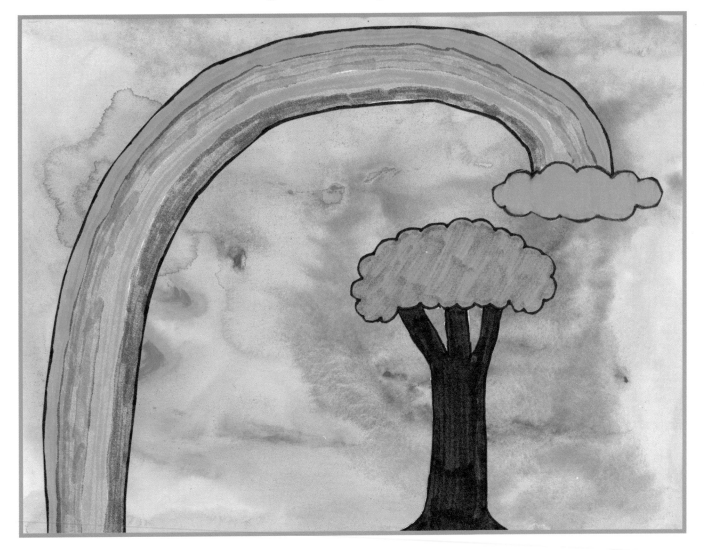

Sometimes Ashley felt as blue as the blue stripe in the rainbow.

Ashley says . . .

" . . . Make sure you show your family you love them! "

Ashley loved her family. Her mom, dad, and brother Kris especially supported and took care of her. She sometimes got angry, but they loved her anyway.

She loved animals too! Ashley had four pets: Angel, Munchkin, and Oscar are the cats and Macho is the dog. She loved them all.

How would you feel if your family helped you through being sick?

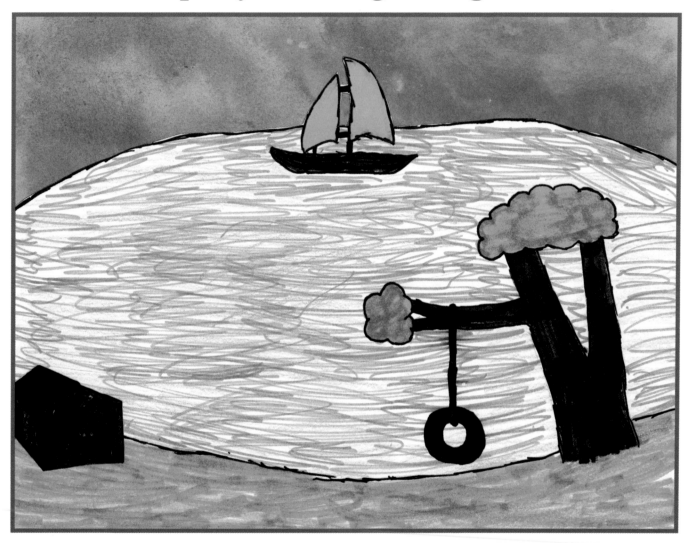

Sometimes Ashley felt as blue as a calm lake.

Ashley says . . .

" . . . Make the most of each moment! "

Being sick didn't stop Ashley from doing what she liked. Jazz dancing, basketball, and soccer were some of her favorite activities. She especially enjoyed playing clarinet in the school band. Ashley had a gigantic collection of Beanie Babies. "Clubby" was her favorite Beanie Baby—he's blue, you know. They even shared the same birth date!

Have you ever felt like you never wanted the day to end?

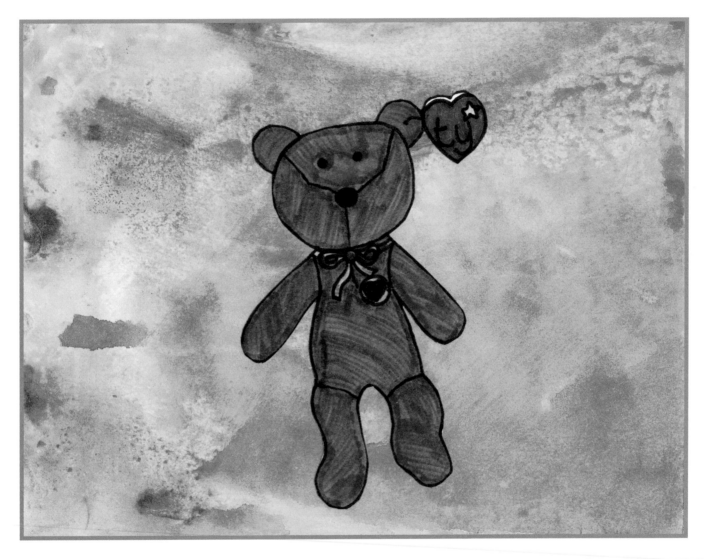

Sometimes Ashley felt as blue as the Beanie Baby "Clubby."

Ashley says . . .

" ... Don't give up! "

Ashley was very healthy the whole summer after her bone marrow transplant. Our class went on a field trip to the zoo on a Friday in September. The following Monday, Ashley wasn't in school. She was sick again. Ashley had a head full of brown hair, but when she came in on Tuesday, *it was all gone*! She told the class, "I had my daddy shave it off. I'm just going to lose it all anyway." No one could believe what they had just heard.

As more time passed, the cancer in her lung got bigger. And bigger.

How would you feel if you thought you were better, but found out the cancer came back?

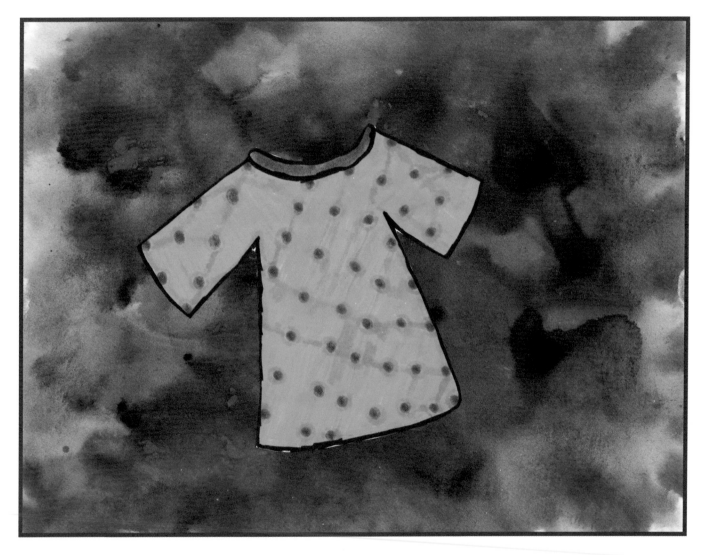

Sometimes Ashley felt as blue as a hospital gown.

Ashley says . . .

" ... Don't be afraid to try new things! "

Being sick meant wearing hats again—not that Ashley didn't like wearing hats. She loved wearing hats, but being the only one wearing them didn't seem to make her too happy. Then one day, she found a solution to not being the only one wearing something on her head. BANDANNAS! She would wear bandannas to school instead of hats. Her idea was a huge success! Everyone loved her bandanna, and other people started wearing them too.

As time went on, Ashley missed more and more school. Her empty desk was a reminder that she was sick.

How would you feel if you set a fashion trend?

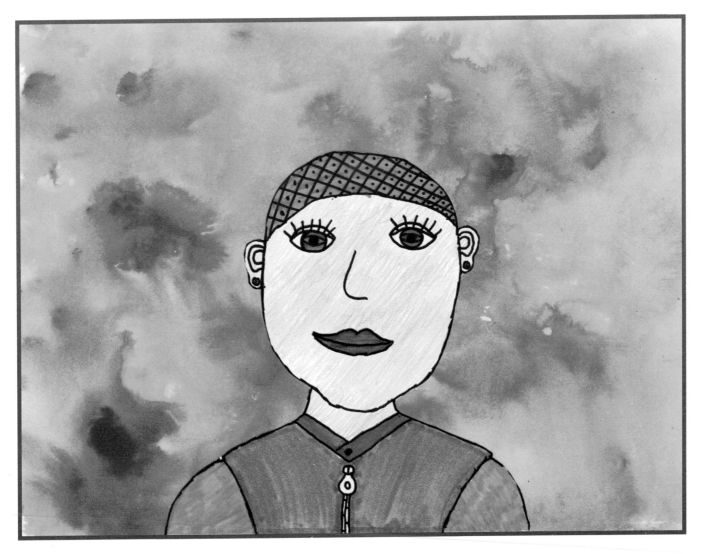

Sometimes Ashley felt as blue as her blue bandanna.

Ashley says. . .

" . . . Don't be blue; I'm still with you! "

Ashley was ten when she died on December 29, 1999. She was watching cartoons with her dad. She looked up at him and he said, "Don't be afraid, it's okay." Then she let go.

How would you feel if you lost someone you love?

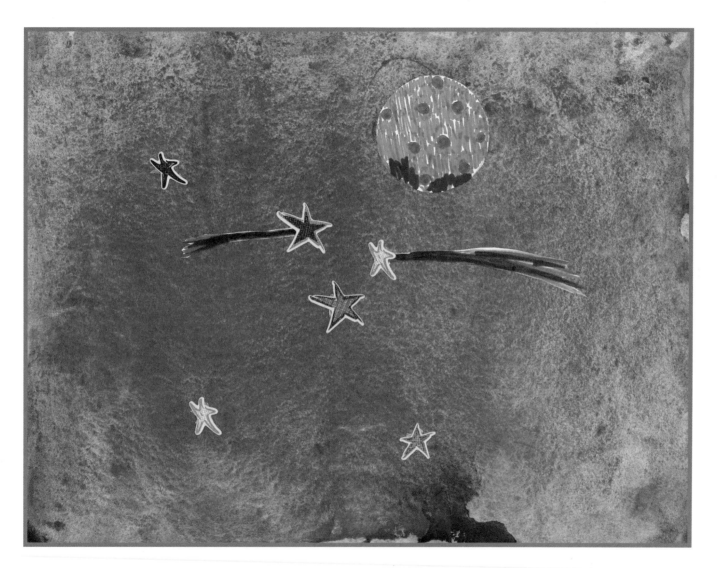

We all feel as blue as the night sky.

Ashley says . . .

" . . . I'm glad I'm a tie-dye angel! "

Ashley's story means many different things to many different people—courage, sadness, hope, faith, life, love, laughter, tears, peace, friendship, happiness, spirit, fun, joy, strength . . . .

Just as in her favorite Backstreet Boys song, "Larger Than Life," Ashley's spirit is still here, larger than life.

We think most Angels dress in white, but Ashley is OUR Angel in BLUE.

How would it feel to be an Angel?

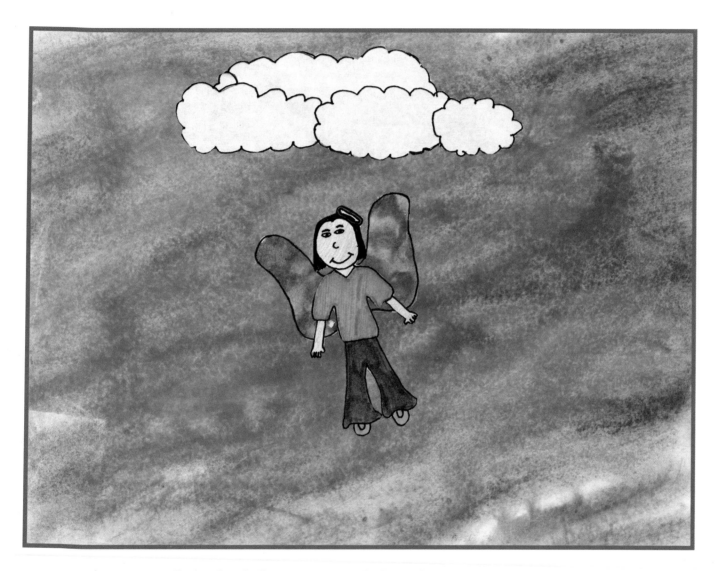

Which blue would YOU choose?

Kids Are Authors®

Books written by children for children

The Kids Are Authors® Competition was established in 1986 to encourage children to read and to become involved in the creative process of writing. Since then, thousands of children have written and illustrated books as participants in the Kids Are Authors® Competition. The winning books in the annual competition are published by Scholastic Inc. and are distributed by Scholastic Book Fairs throughout the United States.

For more information:

Kids Are Authors®
Scholastic Book fairs
PO Box 958411
Lake Mary, FL 32795-8411

Or visit our Web site at
www.scholasticbookfairs.com